ILEOSTOMY DIET

COOKBOOK

Essential Recipes For Post-Surgery Recovery, Nutrient-Rich Meals, Gut Health Maintenance, Digestive Health And More – All You Need To Know

DR. AMARI VALERIE

TABLE OF CONTENTS

BONUS:

7 days meal plan recipes, ingredients, and detailed preparatory guidelines for Ileostomy Diet

7 Desserts procedural recipes for Ileostomy Diet and guidelines

7 Smoothies procedural recipes for Ileostomy Diet and guidelines

DISCLAIMER

The information provided in this book, is for educational and informational purposes only and is not intended as medical advice. The content is not a substitute for professional medical advice, diagnosis, or treatment. Always seek the advice of your physician or other qualified health provider with any questions you may have regarding a medical condition. Never disregard professional medical advice or delay in seeking it because of something you have read in this book.

The dietary suggestions and recipes in this book are based on general guidelines and may not be suitable for everyone. Individual responses to foods can vary, and it is important to consult with a healthcare professional before making any significant changes to your diet.

The author and publisher of this book do not claim to cure or treat any medical condition. The information provided is based on research and personal experience and is intended to help readers make informed decisions about their diet and health.

Furthermore, I the author do not endorse any specific products, brands, treatments, or services that may be mentioned in this book. Any references to products, services, websites, or organizations are provided for informational purposes only and do not constitute an endorsement or recommendation by the author. The inclusion of such references does not imply any association, sponsorship, or affiliation between the author and the referenced entities.

The recipes and dietary suggestions in this book are designed to be safe and healthful. However, readers should use their own discretion and consult with a healthcare professional when necessary, especially if they have allergies, sensitivities, or other dietary restrictions.

By using this book, you acknowledge and agree that the author and publisher shall not be held liable for any loss or damage, including but not limited to special, incidental, consequential, or other damages, resulting from the use of the information and recipes contained in this book.

ABOUT THIS BOOK

This "ILEOSTOMY DIET COOKBOOK" is a critical resource for individuals who are attempting to navigate the intricacies of life following ileostomy surgery. It offers comprehensive advice on the multifaceted aspects of diet and nutrition that are essential for long-term health and recovery. The introduction establishes the context by delineating the fundamentals of an ileostomy, its varieties, and the diverse reasons for which this surgical procedure may be necessary. It explores the surgical procedure and the critical initial recuperation phase, ensuring that readers are aware of the anticipated outcomes and can mentally and physically prepare themselves.

This book provides a comprehensive examination of the critical role that diet plays in the recovery process following surgery.

It delineates the critical relationship between diet and recovery, underscoring the necessity of initially abstaining from specific foods and incorporating others that facilitate healing. Hydration is emphasized as a fundamental component of recovery, in addition to comprehensive discussions regarding nutritional requirements and the potential necessity of supplementation. This section is essential for establishing the groundwork for a successful recovery voyage.

Practical solutions are provided to resolve the common concerns that ileostomy patients encounter. This book provides strategies for addressing dehydration, identifying and preventing food obstructions, managing output consistency, and addressing flatulence and odor issues.

It also addresses the emotional and psychological adaptations that are associated with living with an ileostomy, offering a comprehensive approach to patient care.

Basic dietary guidelines are provided to facilitate the seamless transition of patients to a new eating regimen. The introduction to a low-residue diet, the progressive reintroduction of fiber, and the significance of portion control and meal frequency are meticulously described. The emphasis is on the monitoring of dietary responses and the thorough digestion of food to ensure that patients can customize their diets to their tolerance levels.

The following kitchen techniques are indispensable for the planning and preparation of meals for ileostomy patients. This section guides the safe management and storage of food, as well as the use of practical tools and appliances. Additionally, it offers suggestions for bulk cooking and freezing meals. Additionally, it instructs readers on how to interpret food labels to prevent the presence of concealed ingredients, thereby simplifying and optimizing the process of meal preparation.

From the transition from hospital food to home-cooked meals to the provision of sample meal plans for the initial weeks, this book offers structured guidance on the initiation of the ileostomy diet. It emphasizes the necessity of monitoring the body's response to novel foods, as well as the significance of hydration and electrolyte balance. Protein-rich foods, energy-providing carbohydrates, healthy lipids, essential vitamins and minerals, and recommended supplements are all thoroughly examined to facilitate recovery.

The recipe sections for breakfast, lunch, dinner, snacks, and small dishes are designed to be both nutritious and readily digestible. Gut-friendly smoothies, oatmeal variations, high-protein egg dishes, and straightforward crepes and waffles comprise breakfast recipes. Soups, broths, lean protein dishes, pasta, rice entrees, low-residue salads, and vegetarian options are among the lunch and supper ideas. Energy-boosting smoothies, simple finger foods, light sandwiches, and healthy desserts are the primary focus of snack recipes. Additionally, they emphasize nutritious, easily digestible options.

The primary focus is on the preservation of gastrointestinal health, which includes the exploration of probiotic and prebiotic foods, the reintroduction of fiber, the implementation of hydration strategies, and the resolution of common digestive issues. This book teaches readers how to identify the indications of good versus poor digestive health and offers actionable steps to maintain optimal digestion.

The comprehensive coverage of dining out and social situations includes advice on how to make safe dining decisions, communicate dietary requirements, manage social events, and make informed menu choices. Social participation is not restricted by dietary restrictions due to the availability of portable meals and refreshment ideas.

A dedicated chapter is dedicated to the resolution of common FAQs and troubleshooting, which assists patients in the management of output consistency, the prevention of food blockages, the management of gas and odor issues, the identification of symptoms of dehydration, and the navigation of unanticipated dietary challenges.

This "ILEOSTOMY DIET COOKBOOK" is a comprehensive and supportive resource for individuals who are transitioning to life with an ileostomy. It includes a 7-day meal plan, dessert recipes, and smoothie recipes, ensuring that they can maintain a healthy and satisfying diet following their surgery.

CHAPTER ONE

Introduction

An ileostomy is a surgical procedure that involves the formation of a fistula in the abdomen to facilitate the expulsion of waste from the body when the lower portion of the digestive system is not functioning correctly. This guide provides a comprehensive examination of the ileostomy procedure, including its definition, types, indications, surgical procedures, and initial recovery period.

Comprehending The Ileostomy

The extremity or loop of the small intestine (the ileum) is brought out onto the epidermis to create a surgical opening known as an ileostomy. Its primary function is to facilitate the passage of fecal matter through the stoma, bypassing the colon, rectum, and anus. This procedure is frequently required for patients with conditions such as Crohn's disease, ulcerative colitis, or colorectal cancer, in which the lower digestive tract must be bypassed to ensure optimal waste elimination.

Ileostomy Types

The two primary forms of ileostomies are the end ileostomy and the loop ileostomy. The ileum is taken out through the abdominal wall in an end ileostomy, which entails the removal or bypass of the entire colon.

The stoma is formed by drawing a loop of the ileum out, while a portion of the intestine remains intact. This procedure is known as a loop ileostomy and can be either temporary or permanent. The decision between the two is contingent upon the patient's specific medical condition and surgical objectives.

Justifications For The Need For An Ileostomy

An ileostomy may be necessary for a variety of reasons, such as chronic inflammatory bowel diseases like Crohn's disease and ulcerative colitis, colorectal cancer, congenital defects, trauma, or severe bowel obstructions.

An ileostomy is a critical alternative for waste elimination when these conditions result in irreparable harm or dysfunction to the large intestine. This procedure enhances the patient's quality of life and prevents the development of additional complications.

An Overview Of The Surgical Process

The procedure for establishing an ileostomy typically entails a planned, significant abdominal surgery performed under general anesthesia. The surgeon creates a stoma by making an incision in the abdomen, bringing the ileum through the abdominal wall, and securing it. If the ileostomy is temporary, the rectum is either connected to the ileum or the other end of the intestine is closed. The patient is closely monitored for complications following surgery and is provided with a stoma care plan that outlines the necessary dietary adjustments and stoma management protocols.

The Initial Phase Of Recovery

After an ileostomy, the initial recovery phase entails a hospital stay to facilitate the acquisition of stoma care skills and to monitor the patient. Patients are instructed on the proper methods for cleaning the stoma, changing the ostomy bag, and identifying indicators of complications, such as infection or stoma blockage.

The diet initially comprises clear liquids, which are progressively replaced with low-fiber foods to facilitate digestion. The patient's adaptation to their new lifestyle and the successful recovery of the stoma is guaranteed by routine follow-up visits with the healthcare team.

The Significance Of Diet Following Surgery

The diet is essential for ileostomy patients after surgery, as it facilitates the healing process and assists the digestive system in adapting to its new functioning. Reduced complications, including dehydration and blockages, can be achieved by consuming appropriate foods, which can also enhance overall comfort.

A bland, low-fiber diet is advised immediately following surgery to allow the intestines to recover without irritation. It is imperative to ensure that the body is receiving the essential nutrients while avoiding potential issues by gradually reintroducing foods and monitoring their effects.

The Importance Of Diet In Recovery

The recovery process is significantly influenced by the diet, as it guarantees that the body receives the necessary nutrients for vitality and restoration. It is crucial to consume a well-balanced diet that includes protein for tissue repair, carbohydrates for energy, and healthful lipids.

Digestion can be improved and discomfort can be prevented by consuming small, frequent meals. For example, the body's recovery process can be facilitated by beginning with foods that are readily digestible, such as applesauce, white rice, and lean proteins, which provide mild nourishment without putting undue strain on the digestive system.

Foods To Avoid At First

It is imperative to refrain from consuming specific foods that may result in blockages, flatulence, or irritation following an ileostomy. Initially, it is advisable to refrain from consuming high-fiber foods, including fresh vegetables, nuts, seeds, popcorn, and whole cereals. These foods may be difficult to assimilate and may result in obstructions or discomfort.

Limited consumption of caffeine, carbonated beverages, and spicy foods is also advised, as they have the potential to induce excessive flatulence and irritate the digestive tract.

It is essential to monitor the body's response to various nutrients to determine which ones to gradually reintroduce over time.

Foods That Promote Healing

It is crucial to include foods that are nutrient-rich and simple to assimilate to facilitate healing. Refined cereals, such as white bread and pasta, lean proteins like chicken and fish, peeled fruits, and cooked vegetables are all recommended. These foods offer essential vitamins and minerals without imposing an excessive amount of strain on the digestive system.

For instance, mashed potatoes, scrambled eggs, and creamy peanut butter are excellent choices because they are readily assimilated by the body and are mild on the stomach.

The Significance Of Hydration

The large intestine, which is responsible for water absorption, is bypassed, making hydration especially important for ileostomy patients.

Dehydration is a prevalent issue that can be mitigated by consuming an abundance of fluids. Clear broths, oral rehydration solutions, and water are all viable options for maintaining adequate hydration. Furthermore, the consumption of foods that are hydrating, such as melons, watermelons, and broths, can also contribute to the body's overall hydration. To guarantee consistent hydration, it is advised to consume modest quantities of water throughout the day.

Supplementation And Nutritional Requirements

Ileostomy patients frequently require additional attention to their nutritional intake to guarantee that they are satisfying their body's requirements. Absorption of vitamins and minerals may be compromised as a result of modifications to the digestive system.

Consequently, it may be necessary to supplement with vitamins B12, D, and minerals such as calcium and iron. It is imperative to collaborate with a healthcare provider to monitor blood levels and modify the diet or supplements as necessary. For instance, a daily multivitamin can assist in bridging nutritional deficiencies and promote overall health.

CHAPTER TWO

Common Issues

Following an ileostomy, patients frequently consider the management of their stoma outflow, dietary restrictions, and nutritional balance. To prevent blockages, it is essential to prioritize a well-rounded diet that initially excludes high-fiber foods. While monitoring your body's responses, gradually reintroduce fiber. By maintaining a food diary, you can effectively customize your diet by identifying foods that may cause issues. For example, the consumption of cooked vegetables rather than uncooked ones can facilitate digestion and minimize complications.

Maintaining Consistency In Output

To ensure a consistent output, begin with foods that are readily digestible and low in fiber, such as white grains, pasta, and lean proteins. To regulate stool consistency, gradually introduce small quantities of fiber, such as peeled apples or well-cooked vegetables. If necessary, consume an abundance of fluids and contemplate the use of soluble fiber supplements, such as psyllium husk. To prevent your digestive system from becoming overburdened, consider consuming small, frequent meals and observing the impact of various foods on your output.

Addressing Dehydration

The risk of dehydration is elevated in ileostomy patients as a result of the increased fluid loss. To mitigate this, it is recommended that you consume a minimum of 8-10 containers of fluids per day, which may include clear broths, electrolyte beverages, and water. Consume foods that are hydrating, including soups, cucumbers, and melons. Be attentive to symptoms such as vertigo, parched mouth, or dark urine, and adjust your fluid intake by increasing it. Refrain from consuming alcoholic and caffeine-containing beverages, as they can worsen dehydration.

Identifying Food Obstructions

Initially, prevent food obstructions by digesting food thoroughly and avoiding high-fiber, tough, or stringy foods such as popcorn, nuts, and uncooked vegetables. If you suspect a blockage, symptoms may include abdominal pain, cramping, and decreased output.

It is recommended that you refrain from consuming substantial food and consume tepid fluids. Gently massage your abdomen and walk to encourage movement.

To prevent complications, it is imperative to seek medical attention immediately if symptoms persist for more than a few hours.

Addressing Gas And Odor Concerns

By refraining from consuming foods that are known to induce gas, such as legumes, carbonated beverages, and specific vegetables like broccoli and cabbage, one can reduce the presence of gas and odor. Eat leisurely and refrain from using utensils to minimize air intake. Incorporate odor-reducing foods, such as cranberry juice, parsley, and yogurt, into your diet. Ensure that your appliance is well-fitted to prevent breaches, and use stoma products that are specifically designed to manage odor. Investigate the impact of various foods on flatulence and odor to customize your diet.

Psychological And Emotional Transformations

Seeking assistance from healthcare professionals, support groups, and loved ones is essential for the emotional and psychological adaptation to an ileostomy. Participate in activities that enhance your self-assurance and overall health. To increase your sense of control, it is important to remain informed about your condition. An outlet for your emotions can be achieved by recording your experiences and emotions in a journal. It is common to experience both highs and lows and seeking assistance is a demonstration of strength, not frailty.

CHAPTER THREE

Basic Dietary Recommendations

Individuals with an ileostomy must adhere to fundamental dietary guidelines to preserve their health and prevent complications. At first, concentrate on consuming low-fiber, low-residue foods, including white bread, rice, eggs, and tender proteins, to reduce gastrointestinal activity and prevent blockages.

Reintroduce a diverse selection of foods gradually, ensuring that you consume an adequate amount of fluids to offset the increased water loss caused by the ileostomy. Avoid foods that induce excessive flatulence, odor, or stool thickening, including cabbage, legumes, and carbonated beverages. Maintain a food diary to monitor the foods that are most beneficial for your body and any adverse reactions.

Introduction To A Low-Residue Diet

The objective of a low-residue diet is to minimize the quantity of undigested food that passes through the ileostomy, thereby reducing bowel movements and symptoms of irritation. Easily digestible foods, such as mature bananas, canned fruits, refined cereals, and prepared vegetables without skins or seeds, are included in this diet.

It is advisable to steer clear of high-fiber foods, including whole cereals, unprocessed vegetables, nuts, seeds, and dried fruits, as they have the potential to cause blockages and increase stool volume. The objective is to provide your digestive system with a respite, thereby enabling your stoma to recuperate and function effectively.

The Gradual Reintroduction Of Fiber

Fiber can be gradually reintroduced to your diet after the initial recuperation period on a low-residue diet.

Begin by consuming modest quantities of soluble fiber, which are typically simpler to digest. These fibers are present in foods such as oatmeal, peeled apples, and carrots.

Add additional fiber-rich foods gradually, observing your body's response and discontinuing if you experience any discomfort or changes in stoma output. By maintaining adequate hydration and focusing on a balanced diet that includes both soluble and insoluble fibers, it is possible to gradually increase fiber intake.

Meal Frequency And Portion Control

Eating smaller, more frequent meals is advantageous for individuals with an ileostomy, as it facilitates nutrient assimilation and digestion. Opt for five to six modest meals per day rather than three large ones, as the digestive system may be overburdened. To prevent discomfort and excessive output, it is important to maintain manageable portions. Eat leisurely and chew your food thoroughly to facilitate digestion. This method can assist in the prevention of issues such as swelling and obstructions and the maintenance of consistent energy levels.

The Importance Of Chewing Food Thoroughly

It is essential for individuals with an ileostomy to chew food thoroughly, as it facilitates the digestive process and prevents blockages. Before ingesting, take small nibbles and chew each one until it reaches a smooth consistency. This facilitates the mechanical breakdown of the food, thereby facilitating the absorption and processing of nutrients by your digestive system. Furthermore, the likelihood of larger food particles causing obstructions at the stoma site can be mitigated through the process of thorough digesting. This straightforward practice has the potential to substantially improve the health of your stoma and your overall digestive comfort.

Dietary Monitoring And Adjustment About Individual Tolerance

It is imperative to monitor and alter one's diet to the distinct dietary requirements and tolerances of each individual with an ileostomy. Maintain a comprehensive food diary, documenting the foods you consume and any subsequent symptoms or modifications in stoma output. This can assist in the identification of foods that may induce adverse reactions or discomfort.

Based on these observations, modify your diet by eliminating problematic foods and progressively reintroducing others to assess tolerance.

Consult with a healthcare provider or dietitian regularly to guarantee that your nutritional requirements are satisfactorily addressed while simultaneously managing your ileostomy.

CHAPTER FOUR

Kitchen Suggestions For Patients With Ileostomies

When cooking with an ileostomy, it is advisable to employ silicone implements and non-stick cookware to reduce irritation from harsh scrubbing and minimize cleaning. Utilize a pressure cooker or slow cooker to prepare vegetables and meats that are more easily digestible.

Maintain a food journal to monitor the foods that your body tolerates well and those that cause discomfort. Ileostomy patients need to maintain their hydration by consuming an abundance of fluids while cooking and dining.

Finally, it is advisable to steer clear of high-fiber ingredients, such as seeds and legumes, as they have the potential to cause blockages.

Meal Planning And Preparation

To guarantee a well-balanced diet, devise meals that are high in essential nutrients but low in fiber. Select lean proteins such as poultry, turkey, and fish, and include vegetables that are readily digestible, such as zucchini and carrots. Cook dishes in advance and divide them into portions to alleviate the tension of daily meal preparation and save time. Incorporate carbohydrates that are easily digestible, such as pasta and white rice. To facilitate digestion, it may be beneficial to consume smaller, more frequent meals throughout the day, rather than three substantial ones.

Proper Food Storage And Handling

Always cleanse your hands before handling food to prevent contamination, which is particularly crucial for ileostomy patients who are susceptible to infections. Refrigerate perishable foods at temperatures below 40°F, and freeze them at temperatures below 0°F. Mark remains with the date of preparation and consumes them within three days. To guarantee the safety of the food, it is necessary to reheat it to a minimum of 165°F. To prevent cross-contamination, it is important to keep fresh and cooked foods separate.

Appliances And Instruments That Can Be Beneficial

Invest in a food processor or blender to facilitate the digestion of foods by pureeing them. With minimal effort, a slow cooker or Instant Pot can assist in the preparation of nutrient-rich, tender meals. Utilize a digital kitchen scale to accurately monitor food intake and control portions. Non-stick cookware reduces the necessity for lipids and oils, which can be difficult to digest. Furthermore, a collection of hermetic containers will prevent decomposition and preserve the freshness of the food.

Freezing And Batch Cooking Meals

Batch cooking is a time-saving method for ileostomy patients, enabling them to enjoy nutritious, home-cooked meals with minimal daily effort. Prepare a substantial quantity of soups, stews, and casseroles that can be readily frozen. Label each container with the name and date and use freezer-safe containers.

For the sake of expediency, divide meals into single-serving portions. To reheat, either thaw the dishes in the refrigerator overnight or use the defrost setting on your microwave. To guarantee the safety of foods, they must be adequately heated before consumption.

Uncovering Hidden Ingredients On Food Labels

It is essential to read food labels to prevent the consumption of ingredients that could potentially exacerbate an ileostomy. Be cautious of high-fiber items, artificial sweeteners, and lactose, as they may induce digestive problems. The initial few items are the most important, as the ingredients are enumerated by weight. Products that contain excessive levels of fat and added carbohydrates should be avoided.

Be cautious of ingredients such as chicory root and inulin, which are frequently present in "diet" or "sugar-free" products, as they have the potential to induce bloating and flatulence. Choose foods that contain basic, natural ingredients.

CHAPTER FIVE

Commencing The Ileostomy Diet

It is essential to introduce foods gradually and cautiously when starting the ileostomy diet to enable your digestive system to adapt. Begin with soft, low-fiber foods, including applesauce, bland chicken, white rice, and pears. These nutrients are mild on the digestive system and reduce the likelihood of blockages. To facilitate digestion, consume smaller, more frequent meals and chew your food thoroughly. As your body adjusts, gradually incorporate a greater variety.

Transitioning From Hospital Food To Home-Cooked Meals

The process of transitioning from hospital cuisine to home-cooked meals entails the gradual reintroduction of foods in a controlled manner. To begin, replicate the basic, insipid foods that are served in the hospital, including stewed potatoes, clear broths, and soft-cooked vegetables. Gradually incorporate additional domestic dishes, ensuring that the ingredients and preparation methods are easily digestible. Maintain a food diary to monitor the well-tolerated foods and those that may cause problems.

Foods That Are Both Safe And Easily Digested

White bread, lean meats, smooth peanut butter, and tinned fruits without shells are all safe and simple to digest for ileostomy patients. Initially, it is advisable to refrain from consuming high-fiber foods such as fresh vegetables, nuts, seeds, and peanuts. The digestion of foods can be enhanced through the use of cooking methods such as simmering, heating, and baking.

Furthermore, irritation and discomfort can be mitigated by paring fruits and vegetables and refraining from consuming fiery or highly seasoned foods.

Sample Meal Plans For The Initial Weeks

Meal plans should prioritize digestion and simplicity during the initial weeks. For breakfast, consider incorporating a mature banana into a porridge that is prepared with water or milk. A tiny serving of cooked carrots could accompany a poultry sandwich on white bread for lunch.

For dinner, select steamed green beans, scalloped potatoes, and broiled chicken breast. Plain yogurt or a modest amount of cheese may serve as snacks. These dishes are soothing to the digestive system and provide balanced nutrition.

The Significance Of Electrolyte And Hydration Balance

Ileostomy patients need to maintain electrolyte balance and hydration, as they experience an increase in fluid loss. Consume an abundance of fluids, including electrolyte-rich beverages like sports drinks, medicinal infusions, and water. Incorporate foods that are high in water content, such as melons, watermelon, and soups. If symptoms of dehydration, such as vertigo or dark urine, are observed, oral rehydration solutions may be implemented. It is essential to maintain the balance of electrolytes, particularly sodium and potassium, to prevent complications.

Assessing Your Body's Reaction To Novel Foods

To identify any potential issues, attentively monitor your body's response when introducing new foods. Maintain a comprehensive food diary that includes the foods you consume, the quantities you consume, and any symptoms that may occur, including bloating, pains, or changes in stoma output. This will assist you in identifying foods that may cause distress or obstruction. Introduce one new food at a time to accurately assess tolerance and ensure a balanced, pleasurable diet, gradually increasing the variety and complexity of your diet.

CHAPTER SIX

Essential Nutrients For Recovery

It is imperative to prioritize nutrient-rich foods to facilitate recovery following ileostomy surgery. A balanced diet that includes sufficient protein, carbohydrates, healthy lipids, vitamins, and minerals will facilitate tissue repair, sustain energy levels, and facilitate overall healing. For instance, the body's recovery process is ensured by the inclusion of lean meats, whole cereals, vegetables, and fruits in one's diet.

Protein-Rich Foods That Promote Healing

Proteins are essential for the reconstruction of tissues and the formation of new cells following surgery. Incorporate sources such as lean meats (chicken, poultry), fish, eggs, dairy products (yogurt, cheese), and plant-based options (tofu, lentils). For example, a considerable quantity of protein can be consumed to expedite the healing process, such as a grilled chicken breast served with steamed vegetables or a serving of lentil soup.

Energy From Carbohydrates

The primary energy source and essential for maintaining stamina during recuperation is carbohydrates. Choose complex carbohydrates, including vegetables, fruits, and whole cereals (e.g., porridge, brown rice). A breakfast of oatmeal with fresh berries or a dinner of quinoa and roasted vegetables are excellent examples of how to incorporate healthy carbohydrates into your diet to maintain energy levels.

The Advantages Of Healthy Fats

Healthy lipids are crucial for the reduction of inflammation and the absorption of nutrients. Incorporate sources such as avocados, almonds, seeds, olive oil, and fatty fish (such as mackerel and salmon). For example, a salad that is tossed with olive oil and strewn with chia seeds, or a grilled salmon dish that is served with a side of avocado, can supply the healthy lipids necessary to facilitate recovery.

Minerals And Vitamins That Are Indispensable

Wound healing, immune function, and overall health are contingent upon the presence of vitamins and minerals. Ensure that you consume an adequate amount of vitamin C (citrus fruits, bell peppers), vitamin A (carrots, sweet potatoes), iron (spinach, lean red meat), and zinc (pumpkin seeds, beef).

These essential nutrients can be obtained through a nibble of bell pepper segments with hummus or a meal of spinach salad with lean beef.

Supplements To Consider Following Surgery

Dietary supplements may be required in certain instances to satisfy nutritional requirements following surgery. To address any potential deficiencies, it is advisable to take a multivitamin, and specific supplements such as vitamin D, calcium, and probiotics may be advantageous. Before beginning any new supplements, it is crucial to consult with a healthcare provider to ensure that they are suitable for your unique health requirements.

For example, the maintenance of intestinal health is especially critical following an ileostomy and a daily probiotic supplement can assist in this regard.

CHAPTER SEVEN

Breakfast Recipes

Breakfast preparations that are suitable for individuals with an ileostomy should prioritize nutrient density and ease of digestion. For instance, a creamy banana smoothie can be prepared by blending one ripe banana, one cup of almond milk, one tablespoon of smooth peanut butter, and a teaspoon of honey to add flavor.

Try cinnamon applesauce oatmeal for a warm alternative: cook oats with water or milk, add a tablespoon of applesauce, and sprinkle cinnamon on top. Essential nutrients are provided by high-protein egg dishes, such as scrambled eggs with a side of avocado. For an enjoyable variation, prepare pancakes by combining two pureed bananas with two eggs, cooking them on a non-stick pan, and topping them with a drizzle of maple syrup. Herbal infusions or infused water with cucumber and mint are excellent for maintaining hydration and promoting digestion.

Smoothie Recipes Designed To Promote Gut Health

Smoothies can be a nutritious and easily digestible alternative for individuals with an ileostomy. Blend a cup of coconut water, one banana, half a cucumber, and a fistful of spinach to create a green smoothie that is easy on the intestines. Hydration and fiber are delivered gently by this blend.

Another alternative is a berry yogurt smoothie, which involves blending a cup of plain Greek yogurt with a fistful of mixed berries (strawberries, blueberries, raspberries) and a small amount of almond milk. Gut health is promoted by the antioxidants in the berries and the probiotics in the yogurt. Incorporate a teaspoon of chia seeds that have been steeped in water overnight to provide a calming effect. This can aid indigestion.

Variations Of Oatmeal That Are Simple To Digest

Oatmeal is a breakfast option that is both simple to metabolize and versatile, which is particularly advantageous for individuals with an ileostomy. Consider a banana and honey oatmeal: cook cereals with water or milk until they are creamy, then blend in a spoonful of honey and a mashed banana.

Try pumpkin spice oatmeal for a savory twist: combine cooked oats with a tablespoon of pumpkin purée, a dusting of pumpkin spice, and a small amount of maple syrup. Both variations are mild on the digestive system and offer long-lasting vitality. The nutritional value of the meal can be enhanced and the meal can be more satisfying by serving it with a small amount of almond butter or a few slices of mature avocado to the side.

High-Protein Egg Dishes

Egg dishes that are high in protein are an excellent choice for breakfast, as they provide essential amino acids and vitality. For a straightforward scrambled egg recipe, whisk two eggs with a small amount of milk, prepare them in a non-stick pan with a small amount of butter, and serve them with a side of sliced avocado to provide healthy lipids.

Another option is an egg and spinach scramble: sauté a small amount of baby spinach in olive oil until it is wilted, then add scrambled eggs and simmer until they are set. Not only are these dishes quick and simple to prepare, but they are also mild on the digestive system, making them an ideal choice for individuals who are managing an ileostomy.

Pancakes And Waffles That Are Both Simple And Nutritious

Make straightforward banana pancakes for a nutritious and delectable breakfast: mash one ripe banana, combine with two eggs and cook small pancakes on a non-stick pan until golden brown. These crepes are naturally sweet and simple to digest. Blend one cup of oats into flour, combine with a pureed banana, an egg, and a small amount of milk to form a batter consistency, and cook in a waffle maker.

Both recipes are an ideal choice for a mild and substantial breakfast, as they can be enhanced with a dollop of Greek yogurt and a drizzle of honey to provide additional flavor and nutrition.

Morning Beverages That Are Hydrating

Individuals with an ileostomy need to maintain proper hydration, particularly in the morning. To begin your day, prepare a soothing ginger and lemon tea by steeping fresh ginger segments in hot water, adding a squeeze of lemon, and a hint of honey for sweetness.

An additional alternative is cucumber mint water, which involves infusing a container of water with fresh mint leaves and cucumber segments in the refrigerator overnight. These hydrating beverages not only promote fluid balance but also offer a revitalizing start to the day, thereby promoting overall digestion and well-being.

CHAPTER EIGHT

Ideas For Lunch And Dinner

Concentrate on dishes that are easily digestible and gentle on the digestive system for lunch and evening.

A nutritious, low-fiber entrée can be prepared by grilling a chicken breast and serving it with steamed vegetables and mashed potatoes. A broiled white fish with sautéed vegetables and a side of quinoa is a nutritious meal that does not overtax the digestive system.

An additional alternative is a poultry meatloaf that is accompanied by a creamy polenta and green asparagus. The objective of these meals is to reduce digestive distress while maintaining nutritional value.

Soups And Broths That Are Easily Digestible

The soothing nature and simplicity of assimilation of soups and broths make them an excellent choice for ileostomy patients. A comforting option is a traditional poultry broth that is flavored with finely diced vegetables such as celery, carrots, and potatoes. Pureed vegetable soups, including butternut squash soup and smooth tomato basil soup, are both delightful and easy on the digestive system. Bone broth can be incorporated into these soups to enhance their nutritional value, thereby ensuring that they are easily digestible and contain essential vitamins and minerals.

Vegetable-Based Lean Protein Dishes

Meals that are both nutritious and gratifying are achieved by combining well-cooked vegetables with lean proteins. Attempt a roasted salmon entrée with a serving of steamed zucchini and mashed sweet potatoes. An alternative concept is a grilled turkey patty that is served without a bun, accompanied by a small portion of white rice and sautéed bell peppers. These dishes are designed to support the overall health of ileostomy patients and facilitate the digestion process by providing essential protein and minerals.

Suitable Ileostomy Patient Meals: Pasta And Rice

Pasta and rice dishes are excellent choices for ileostomy patients, as they are typically simple to metabolize and can be prepared with low-fiber ingredients.

A straightforward pasta dish that is both flavorful and easy on the stomach is accompanied by soft-cooked chicken segments and a buttery alfredo sauce. In contrast, a risotto prepared with Arborio rice, chicken broth, and finely minced mushrooms offers a creamy, nutritious entrée. These dishes provide a gratifying culinary experience while ensuring that the digestive system is not overburdened.

Salads With Minimal Waste

Salads can be altered to be low-residue and appropriate for patients with ileostomies. A cucumber and avocado salad with a mild yogurt vinaigrette is a classic example. Another alternative is a caprese salad, which is prepared by serving sliced tomatoes, fresh mozzarella, and basil with a sprinkling of olive oil.

To create a more substantial salad, combine cooked quinoa with diced cucumbers, bell peppers, and a small amount of feta cheese. These salads are intended to be both fresh and nutritious, while also being gentle on the digestive system.

Vegetarian Meals That Are High In Nutrients

Careful ingredient selection can result in vegetarian dishes that are both nutrient-dense and appropriate for ileostomy patients. A lentil broth that is both nourishing and easy on the digestive system is prepared with carrots, potatoes, and well-cooked lentils.

Another alternative is a tofu stir-fry that is accompanied by white rice and soft-cooked vegetables such as zucchini, bell peppers, and snap peas.

These dishes guarantee a balanced diet that promotes overall health and well-being by providing essential nutrients, including protein, vitamins, and minerals.

CHAPTER NINE

Snacks And Small Meals

It is crucial to consume refreshments that are both readily digestible and nutritious when managing an ileostomy. Alternatives such as plain yogurt, applesauce, or pureed bananas are mild on the digestive system. Rice cakes that are lightly distributed with peanut butter or cheese can be both simple to digest and satisfying. Protein-rich foods, such as hard-boiled eggs or hummus with soft pita bread, and soft-cooked vegetables, such as zucchini or carrots, are also excellent choices. Initially, prioritize foods that are low in fiber and progressively introduce higher-fiber options as tolerated.

Smoothies That Increase Energy Levels

Energy-boosting smoothies can offer essential nutrients while being gentle on the digestive system. Combine ingredients such as bananas, mangos, or fruit with a basis of almond milk or lactose-free yogurt. For an additional energy boost, incorporate a tablespoon of protein powder or a teaspoon of peanut butter. Initially, it is advisable to steer clear of seeds and high-fiber ingredients; instead, opt for smooth and creamy alternatives. For instance, a smoothie that contains spinach, banana, avocado, and almond milk is an excellent choice, as it delivers vitamins and healthy lipids without irritating.

Appetizers And Finger Foods That Are Simple

Finger foods and appetizers that are simple in nature should be both pleasurable and mild on the digestive system. Soft cheese cubes, small segments of turkey or poultry, and peeled cucumber slices can be used to create simple and delectable treats.

Initially, it is advisable to steer clear of fresh vegetables with seeds or tough shells. Soft avocado slices, deviled eggs, and mild cheese and cracker combinations are also excellent options. These items are not only palatable but also easily digestible, rendering them an excellent choice for individuals with ileostomies.

Sandwiches And Wraps That Are Light In Weight

Individuals with an ileostomy may find light sandwiches and wraps to be both convenient and appropriate. Use soft, white bread or tortillas to create sandwiches with lean proteins such as turkey or chicken. For added flavor, apply a thin layer of mayonnaise or mustard.

Incorporate fillings that are readily digestible, such as cheese, avocado, or peeled cucumber. Opt for silky textures and steer clear of high-fiber ingredients.

A balanced meal that is easy on the digestive system can be achieved by incorporating a small amount of lettuce (without stiff stems) into a basic turkey and cheese wrap.

Healthy Dessert Alternatives

Soft, readily consumable desserts are viable alternatives for an ileostomy diet. Serve apples or pears with a dusting of cinnamon after baking them until they are tender. Desserts that are smooth and velvety, such as vanilla pudding, rice pudding, or gelatin-based delights, can also be satisfying.

If you prefer a chilled delight, consider lactose-free sorbet or ice cream that is prepared from smooth, pureed fruits. To guarantee that the confection is mild on your digestive system, refrain from incorporating nuts, seeds, and high-fiber ingredients.

CHAPTER TEN

Preserving Gut Health

Individuals with an ileostomy need to maintain intestinal health, as it can help prevent complications and ensure overall well-being. This entails the integration of foods that are readily digestible into the diet, including lean proteins, prepared vegetables, and soft fruits.

It is also crucial to refrain from consuming foods that may cause irritation or obstructions, such as raw vegetables, nuts, and tough proteins. Furthermore, digestion and discomfort can be mitigated by consuming small, frequent meals and digesting food thoroughly. Maintaining a food diary to monitor any reactions or symptoms can assist in the identification of trigger foods and the optimization of digestive health.

Foods That Contain Probiotics And Prebiotics

The development of beneficial bacteria can be facilitated by the inclusion of probiotic and prebiotic foods in the diet, which can support digestive health. Yogurt, kefir, and fermented vegetables such as sauerkraut and kimchi are all examples of probiotic nutrients.

Furthermore, these foods introduce live cultures of beneficial bacteria into the intestines, which can assist in the preservation of a healthy balance of microorganisms. Bananas, scallions, and garlic are examples of prebiotic foods that contain fibers that contribute to the growth and activity of beneficial microbes. Supporting digestive health and overall well-being can be achieved by incorporating a diverse selection of probiotic and prebiotic foods into one's diet.

Fiber: When And How To Reintroduce It

It is important to progressively reintroduce fiber into the diet after ileostomy surgery to prevent digestive discomfort or obstructions. Proceed with caution. To begin, incorporate low-fiber foods, including white bread, white grains, and peeled fruits, and progressively increase fiber intake over time.

The digestive system should be given time to acclimate to high-fiber foods, such as raw vegetables, legumes, and whole cereals, by introducing them gradually and in small quantities.

It is imperative to consume an abundance of water when increasing fiber intake to prevent constipation and facilitate digestion. Individuals can achieve the optimal balance for their digestive health by monitoring their gastrointestinal movements and modifying their fiber intake accordingly.

Strategies For Optimizing Digestion: Hydration

Individuals with an ileostomy must maintain optimal digestion and prevent dehydration by staying hydrated. Replacing fluids lost through stoma output can be achieved by consuming an abundance of fluids throughout the day, such as water, medicinal infusions, and electrolyte-rich beverages.

Dehydration and digestive system irritation may result from the consumption of sugary or caffeinated beverages. Therefore, it is crucial to refrain from consuming them. Monitoring urine color and discharge can assist in determining hydration levels, with pale yellow urine suggesting that the individual is adequately hydrated.

Drinking fluids regularly and transporting a water bottle can help guarantee optimal digestion and consistent hydration.

Handling Typical Digestive Problems

It is imperative for individuals with an ileostomy to address common digestive issues, including bloating, flatulence, and diarrhea, to preserve their comfort and overall health. Symptoms can be alleviated by refraining from trigger foods, including dairy products, carbonated beverages, and piquant foods.

Digestion can be facilitated and discomfort can be reduced by consuming small, frequent meals and digesting food completely. Preventing digestive issues can be achieved by incorporating readily digestible foods into the diet, including cooked vegetables, lean proteins, and soft fruits.

Individuals can effectively manage their digestive health by maintaining a food diary to monitor symptoms and identify trigger foods.

If you are experiencing persistent digestive issues, it is advisable to consult with a healthcare professional for personalized advice and support.

CHAPTER ELEVEN

Social Situations And Dining Out

Eating out can be a daunting experience for individuals with an ileostomy; however, with the assistance of a few smart strategies, it can be a stress-free and enjoyable experience. Ensure that you review the menu online in advance to identify secure choices, such as grilled chicken or seafood, steamed vegetables, and rice.

Do not hesitate to inform the server of your dietary restrictions when placing an order. For instance, to regulate one's consumption, it is advisable to request condiments and dressings on the side and steer clear of dishes that are excessively oily or spicy, as they may induce digestive issues. If the primary dishes appear to be excessively large, consider ordering lesser portions or appetizers.

In the event of an emergency, it is advisable to discreetly transport a small supply of ostomy supplies in your purse. Do not allow your ileostomy to restrict your social life; rather, employ these strategies to confidently navigate dining out.

Ideas For Portable Meals And Snacks

It is essential to be equipped with portable meals and refreshment options to regulate appetite and maintain energy levels throughout the day. For on-the-go snacks, bring foods that are easily digestible, such as bananas, yogurt, rice cakes, and nut butter sachets.

For meals, contemplate constructing sandwiches with soft, readily digestible fillings, such as scrambled eggs or tuna salad. Pre-cut fruits and vegetables, such as carrots, pears, and cucumber segments, are both nutritious and convenient.

Invest in a quality insulated picnic bag to keep perishable items fresh, and always carry extra ostomy supplies just in case. These portable alternatives enable you to sustain a nutritious diet and remain content regardless of your daily activities.

Suggestions For Eating Out Safely

It is imperative to prioritize food safety when dining out to prevent potential complications with your ileostomy. Select establishments that are known for their clean facilities and their commitment to the proper management of food. When placing an order, prioritize dishes that are readily digestible and well-cooked, such as grilled or baked proteins, steamed vegetables, and simple rice or pasta.

It is advisable to steer clear of raw or undercooked foods, as they may be more difficult to digest and may increase the likelihood of bacterial contamination. Please notify your server of your dietary restrictions and inquire about the ingredients or preparation methods if you are uncertain. You can dine out safely and worry-free by being proactive and selective in your choices.

Making Informed Decisions On The Menu

A strategic approach is necessary to ensure optimal digestion and minimal distress when navigating restaurant menus with an ileostomy. Select menu items that are low in fiber and cholesterol, as these can be more difficult to digest and may result in digestive issues.

Select lean protein sources, such as chicken, fish, or tofu, and combine them with basic carbohydrates, such as rice or potatoes, and well-cooked vegetables. Dishes that contain hefty sauces, spicy seasonings, or excessive quantities of dairy should be avoided, as they may exacerbate digestive symptoms. Alternatively, select seared or steamed dishes and request that they be adjusted to accommodate your dietary requirements. You can savor delectable meals without sacrificing your digestive health by making informed menu selections.

Communicating Dietary Requirements To Others

Ensuring a comfortable dining experience with an ileostomy necessitates effectively communicating your dietary requirements to restaurant staff, friends, and family. Be forthright and forthright regarding your dietary restrictions, providing a rationale for your decisions if required.

It is crucial to provide loved ones with explicit instructions when they are preparing meals, emphasizing the significance of avoiding trigger foods or ingredients.

Do not hesitate to inquire about the menu options or request modifications to suit your requirements when dining out.

A dietary card or note that outlines your restrictions should be carried with you to present to stewards or chefs if necessary. You can confidently navigate social situations and appreciate meals without concern by communicating assertively and advocating for yourself.

CHAPTER TWELVE

7-Day Meal Plan Ingredients And Detailed Preparatory Guidelines For Ileostomy Diet

DAY ONE:

Breakfast:

Smooth Banana Oatmeal

INGREDIENTS:

• One cup of rolled oats

• Two pints of water

• One pureed mature banana

• One tablespoon of honey

• 1/2 teaspoon of cinnamon

PREPARATION:

1. Bring water to a simmer in a vessel.

2. Add grains and reduce the heat to a simmer.

3. Stir intermittently during the 5-minute cooking period.

4. Mix in honey, cinnamon, and pureed banana.

5. Arrange for a heated serving.

Snack:

Apple sauce

INGREDIENTS:

• Four apples, trimmed and sliced

• One cup of water

• One tablespoon of sugar

• 1/2 teaspoon of cinnamon

PREPARATION:

1. Combine all ingredients in a saucepan.

2. Cook the pears over medium heat until they are tender.

3. Blend or mash until the desirable consistency is achieved.

4. Chill before serving.

Lunch:

Chicken and Rice Soup

INGREDIENTS:

• One prepared and diced chicken breast

• One-half cup of prepared white rice

• Four pints of poultry broth

• One carrot, trimmed and diced

• One celery stalk, sliced

• Salt to flavor

PREPARATION:

1. Bring bouillon to a simmer in a pot.

2. Mix in the carrot and celery, and sauté until they are soft.

3. Incorporate prepared rice and shredded chicken.

4. Simmer for 5-10 minutes.

5. Mix in salt and serve while still warm.

Snack:

Honey and Greek Yogurt

INGREDIENTS:

• One cup of Greek yogurt

• One tablespoon of honey

PREPARATION:

1. Combine honey with Greek yogurt.

2. Chill before serving.

INGREDIENTS:

• One salmon tenderloin

• Two potatoes, skinned and sliced

• Two tablespoons of olive oil

• Salt and pepper to flavor

PREPARATION:

1. Turn the oven on to 375°F, or 190°C.

2. Place the salmon on a baking sheet, drizzle with 1 tablespoon of olive oil, and season with salt and pepper.

3. Bake for 20 minutes or until the food is fully finished.

4. Mash potatoes with the remaining olive oil, salt, and pepper after boiling them until they are tender.

5. Serve salmon with boiled potatoes.

Juice:

Apple and Carrot Juice

INGREDIENTS:

• Two carrots, peeled

• Two apples, trimmed and cored

• One cup of water

PREPARATION:

1. All ingredients should be blended until they are homogeneous.

2. If desirable, strain the mixture.

3. Chill before serving.

DAY TWO:

INGREDIENTS:

- Two eggs

- One half of an avocado, divided

- One tablespoon of butter

- Salt to flavor

PREPARATION:

1. In a basin, beat eggs with a sprinkle of salt.

2. Melt butter in a saucepan over medium heat.

3. Gently stir the eggs in the pan until they are scrambled.

4. Accompany the dish with diced avocado on the side.

Snack:

Sauce made from pears

INGREDIENTS:

• Four pears, skinned and sliced

• One cup of water

• One tablespoon of sugar

PREPARATION:

1. In a saucepan, combine sugar, water, and pears.

2. Cook the pears over medium heat until they are tender.

3. Blend or mash until the desirable consistency is achieved.

4. Chill before serving.

Creamy Pumpkin Soup

INGREDIENTS:

• Two cups of pumpkin puree

• Two quarts of poultry broth

• 1/2 cup of coconut milk

• 1/2 teaspoon of powdered ginger

• Salt to flavor

PREPARATION:

1. Combine ground ginger, chicken broth, and pumpkin purée in a saucepan.

2. Bring the mixture to a simmer and allow it to cook for a duration of 10 minutes.

3. Add salt and coconut milk to flavor.

4. Arrange for a heated serving.

Rice crackers topped with cheese

INGREDIENTS:

• Ten rice crackers

• Cottage cheese, 1/2 cup

PREPARATION:

1. Apply cottage cheese to rice wafers.

2. Serve immediately.

Dinner:

Rice and Turkey Meatballs

INGREDIENTS:

• One pound of minced turkey

• One egg

• 1/4 cup of breadcrumbs

- 1/4 cup of grated Parmesan cheese

- One tablespoon of olive oil

- One cup of prepared white rice

- Salt and pepper to flavor

PREPARATION:

1. Preheat the oven to 375°F (190°C).

2. Combine minced turkey, egg, breadcrumbs, Parmesan cheese, salt, and pepper in a basin.

3. Shape the mixture into meatballs and arrange them on a baking sheet.

4. Bake for 20 minutes and drizzle with olive oil.

5. Serve meatballs with prepared white rice.

Ginger and Pear Juice

INGREDIENTS:

• Two pears, trimmed and cored

• One small piece of ginger, trimmed

• One cup of water

PREPARATION:

1. All ingredients should be blended until they are homogeneous.

2. If desirable, strain the mixture.

3. Chill before serving.

THIRD DAY:

Breakfast:

Smoothie with blueberries

INGREDIENTS:

• One cup of blueberries

• One banana

• One-half cup of Greek yogurt

• One-half cup of almond milk

PREPARATION:

1. All ingredients should be blended until they are homogeneous.

2. Serve immediately.

Snack:

Banana Bread

INGREDIENTS:

• Two mature bananas, pureed

• 1/4 cup of sugar

• 1/4 cup of molten butter

• One egg

• One cup of flour

• One teaspoon of baking soda

• 1/4 teaspoon of salt

PREPARATION:

1. Set the oven's temperature to 175°C/350°F.

2. In a basin, combine the pureed bananas, sugar, butter, and egg.

3. Mix in the flour, baking soda, and salt.

4. Pour the batter into a loaf pan that has been greased.

5. Bake for 60 minutes or until a toothpick inserted into the center of the cake emerges clean.

6. Allow to cool before serving.

Lunch:

Chicken and Avocado Salad

INGREDIENTS:

• One roasted and cut chicken breast

• One avocado, minced

• 1/4 cup of cherry tomatoes, halved

• One tablespoon of olive oil

• One tablespoon of lemon juice

• Salt and pepper to flavor

PREPARATION:

1. Combine chicken, avocado, and cherry tomatoes in a basin.

2. Drizzle with lemon juice and olive oil.

3. Add salt and pepper to taste.

4. Serve immediately.

Snack:

Hummus and Cucumber Slices

INGREDIENTS:

• One cucumber, sliced

• 1/2 cup of hummus

PREPARATION:

1. Serve cucumber segments with tahini for dipping.

Dinner:

Steamed Carrots with Baked Cod

INGREDIENTS:

• One cod fillet

• Two carrots, trimmed and cut

• One tablespoon of olive oil

• Salt and pepper to flavor

PREPARATION:

1. Preheat the oven to 375°F (190°C).

2. Place the cod on a baking sheet, drizzle with olive oil, and season with salt and pepper.

3. Bake for 15-20 minutes or until the food is fully cooked.

4. Steam carrots until they are soft.

5. Steamed vegetables should be served alongside halibut.

Juice:

Strawberry Banana Juice

INGREDIENTS:

• One cup of hulled strawberries

• One banana

• One cup of water

PREPARATION:

1. All ingredients should be blended until they are homogeneous.

2. If desirable, strain the mixture.

3. Chill before serving.

DAY FOUR:

INGREDIENTS:

• One cup of prepared white rice

• One cup of milk

• Two tablespoons of sugar

• 1/2 teaspoon of vanilla extract

PREPARATION:

1. Combine cooked rice, milk, sugar, and vanilla in a saucepan.

2. Cook over medium heat until the mixture thickens, which should take approximately 15 minutes.

3. Serve either at room temperature or refrigerated.

Smoothie with peaches

INGREDIENTS:

• One peach, skinned and cut

• One-half cup of Greek yogurt

• One-half cup of almond milk

• One tablespoon of honey

PREPARATION:

1. All ingredients should be blended until they are homogeneous.

2. Serve immediately.

INGREDIENTS:

• Two cups of butternut squash, trimmed and diced

• One carrot, trimmed and diced

• Four pints of poultry broth

• 1/2 cup of coconut milk

• Salt to flavor

PREPARATION:

1. Butternut squash, carrot, and poultry broth should be combined in a saucepan.

2. Bring the mixture to a boil, then reduce the heat and allow it to simmer until the vegetables are soft.

3. The soup should be blended until it is smooth.

4. Add salt and coconut milk. Stir.

5. Arrange for a heated serving.

Snack:

Soft-boiled eggs

INGREDIENTS:

• Two eggs

• Salt to flavor

PREPARATION:

1. Water is brought to a boil in a container.

2. Gently lower eggs into simmering water.

3. Continue to cook for six minutes.

4. Eggs should be removed and cooled in cold water.

5. Peel and serve with a sprinkle of salt.

INGREDIENTS:

• One pound of minced turkey

• Two bowls of mashed potatoes

• One-half cup of chicken bouillon

• One carrot, trimmed and diced

• 1/2 cup of peas

• One tablespoon of olive oil

• Salt and pepper to flavor

PREPARATION:

1. Turn the oven on to 375°F, or 190°C.

2. Cook ground turkey in a pan with olive oil until it is browned.

3. Add carrots, peas, and chicken broth; cook until the vegetables are soft.

4. Transfer the mixture to a baking dish and sprinkle with pureed potatoes.

5. Bake for 20 minutes or until the top is a golden brown color.

6. Arrange for a heated serving.

Juice:

Melon Mint Juice

INGREDIENTS:

• Two cups of diced and trimmed melon

• One tablespoon of fresh mint fronds

• One cup of water

PREPARATION:

1. All ingredients should be blended until they are homogeneous.

2. If desirable, strain the mixture.

3. Chill before serving.

DAY FIVE:

Breakfast:

Berry Yogurt Parfait

INGREDIENTS:

• One cup of Greek yogurt

• 1/2 cup of assorted berries (strawberries, raspberries, and blueberries)

• One tablespoon of honey

PREPARATION:

1. Arrange Greek yogurt, honey, and berries in a glass.

2. Serve immediately.

Snack:

Mango Smoothie

INGREDIENTS:

• One mango, skinned and minced

• One-half cup of Greek yogurt

• One-half cup of almond milk

PREPARATION:

1. All ingredients should be blended until they are homogeneous.

2. Serve immediately.

Tuna and Avocado Salad

INGREDIENTS:

• One tuna can, drained

• Diced half of an avocado

• 1/4 cup of cherry tomatoes, halved

• One tablespoon of olive oil

• One tablespoon of lemon juice

• Salt and pepper to flavor

PREPARATION:

1. Combine cherry tomatoes, avocado, and tuna in a basin.

2. Drizzle with lemon juice and olive oil.

3. Add salt and pepper to taste.

4. Serve immediately.

Snack:

Carrot sticks with ranch dip

INGREDIENTS:

• Two carrots, peeled and split into spears

• 1/2 cup of ranch dip

PREPARATION:

1. Present carrot spears with ranch dressing for dipping.

Dinner:

Recipe for Baked Chicken with Quinoa

INGREDIENTS:

• One chicken breast

• 1/2 cup of quinoa

• One cup of chicken bouillon

• One tablespoon of olive oil

• Salt and pepper to flavor

PREPARATION:

1. Preheat the oven to 375°F (190°C).

2. Place the chicken on a baking sheet, drizzle with olive oil, and season with salt and pepper.

3. Bake for 20-25 minutes or until the food is fully cooked.

4. In the interim, prepare the quinoa in chicken broth according to the instructions on the container.

5. Quinoa should be served alongside roasted poultry.

Orange and Pineapple Juice

INGREDIENTS:

• One cup of minced and trimmed pineapple

• One orange, skinned and segmented

• One cup of water

PREPARATION:

1. All ingredients should be blended until they are homogeneous.

2. If desirable, strain the mixture.

3. Chill before serving.

DAY SIX:

Apple Cinnamon Pancakes

INGREDIENTS:

• One cup of flour

• One tablespoon of sugar

• One teaspoon of baking powder

• 1/2 teaspoon of cinnamon

• One egg

• One cup of milk

• One apple, peeled and grated

PREPARATION:

1. Combine cinnamon, sugar, baking powder, and flour in a basin.

2. Beat the egg and milk in a separate basin.

3. Combine the dry ingredients with the liquid ingredients until they are barely combined.

4. Gently incorporate the grated apple.

5. Cook pancakes over medium heat on a greased griddle until they are golden brown.

6. Arrange for a heated serving.

Snack:

Crackers and soft cheese

INGREDIENTS:

• Ten rice crackers

• 1/2 cup of mild cheese (e.g., camembert or brie)

PREPARATION:

1. Soft cheese should be served with rice crackers.

INGREDIENTS:

• Two cups of broccoli florets

• One potato, skinned and minced

• Four pints of poultry broth

• 1/2 cup of coconut milk

• Salt to flavor

PREPARATION:

1. Combine broccoli, potato, and chicken bouillon in a saucepan.

2. Bring the mixture to a boil, then reduce the heat and allow it to simmer until the vegetables are soft.

3. The soup should be blended until it is smooth.

4. Add salt and coconut milk. Stir.

5. Arrange for a heated serving.

Snack:

Slices of melon

INGREDIENTS:

• One cup of cut and trimmed melon

PREPARATION:

1. Chill the melon segments before serving.

Dinner:

Stir-Fry of Shrimp and Rice

INGREDIENTS:

• 1/2 pound of shrimp, skinned and deveined

• One cup of prepared white rice

- One carrot, trimmed and diced

- 1/4 cup of legumes

- One tablespoon of olive oil

- One tablespoon of soy sauce

- Salt and pepper to flavor

PREPARATION:

1. Heat olive oil in a pan over medium heat.

2. Add the shrimp and sauté until they are opaque and pink.

3. Stir-fry the carrot, peas, and heated rice for five minutes.

4. Season with salt and pepper and add soy sauce.

5. Arrange for a heated serving.

Juice:

Lemonade with Cucumber

INGREDIENTS:

• One cucumber, trimmed and diced

• Juice from one lemon

• One tablespoon of honey

• One cup of water

PREPARATION:

1. All ingredients should be blended until they are homogeneous.

2. If desirable, strain the mixture.

3. Chill before serving.

SEVENTH DAY:

Breakfast:

Avocado Toast

INGREDIENTS:

• One slice of buttered whole-grain bread

• Mashed half of an avocado

• Salt and pepper to flavor

PREPARATION:

1. Apply pureed avocado to toast.

2. Add salt and pepper to taste.

3. Serve immediately.

Snack:

Banana Smoothie

INGREDIENTS:

• One banana

• One-half cup of Greek yogurt

• One-half cup of almond milk

• One tablespoon of honey

PREPARATION:

1. All ingredients should be blended until they are homogeneous.

2. Serve immediately.

Soup with Basil and Tomatoes

INGREDIENTS:

• Four tomatoes, trimmed and sliced

• One cup of chicken bouillon

• Chopped 1/4 cup of fresh basil leaves

• 1/2 cup of coconut milk

• Salt to flavor

PREPARATION:

1. Combine chicken bouillon and tomatoes in a saucepan.

2. Bring the mixture to a boil, then reduce the heat and allow it to simmer until the tomatoes are tender.

3. The soup should be blended until it is smooth.

4. Combine basil, coconut milk, and salt.

5. Arrange for a heated serving.

Snack:

Soft pretzels

INGREDIENTS:

• One cup of tepid water

• One tablespoon of sugar

• One teaspoon of salt

• 2 1/4 teaspoons of active dried yeast

• Three cups of flour

• 1/4 cup of baking soda

• One pounded egg

PREPARATION:

1. Preheat the oven to 450°F (230°C).

2. Combine sugar, salt, and tepid water in a basin. Sprinkle yeast on the surface and allow it to remain until it becomes frothy.

3. Mix in the flour to create a dough.

4. Knead the dough on a floured surface until it is smooth.

5. Divide the dough into eight equal portions, braid each into a rope, and mold each into a pretzel shape.

6. Add baking soda to 10 glasses of water that has been brought to a boil. Boil pretzels in batches for 30 seconds each.

7. Place the pretzels on a baking sheet, cover them with beaten egg, and bake them for 12-15 minutes.

8. Arrange for a heated serving.

Dinner:

Green Beans and Baked Tilapia

INGREDIENTS:

• One fillet of tilapia

• One cup of trimmed green beans

• One tablespoon of olive oil

• Salt and pepper to flavor

PREPARATION:

1. Preheat the oven to 375°F (190°C).

2. Place the tilapia on a baking sheet, drizzle with olive oil, and season with salt and pepper.

3. Bake for 15-20 minutes or until the food is fully cooked.

4. Green beans should be steamed until they are soft.

5. Green legumes should be served alongside tilapia.

Juice:

Watermelon Mint Juice

INGREDIENTS:

• Two cups of minced and peeled melons

• One tablespoon of fresh mint fronds

• One cup of water

PREPARATION:

1. All ingredients should be blended until they are homogeneous.

2. If desirable, strain the mixture.

3. Chill before serving.

This seven-day meal plan for an ileostomy diet comprises breakfast, lunch, dinner, snacking, and juice recipes that are both nutritious and easily digestible.

CHAPTER THIRTEEN

Seven Dessert Procedural Recipes For Ileostomy Diet

Careful consideration of diet is necessary to ensure proper digestion and nutrient assimilation while living with an ileostomy. This compendium offers seven delectable dessert recipes that are specifically designed for individuals with an ileostomy. The emphasis of these recipes is on the use of ingredients that are easily digestible, low in fiber, and free of potential impediments. Guidelines for maintaining a balanced and pleasant diet are included with each recipe.

1. BANANA PUDDING

INGREDIENTS:

• Three fully mature avocados

• One cup of vanilla yogurt

• One tablespoon of honey

• One teaspoon of vanilla extract

STEPS:

1. In a basin, mash the bananas until they are pureed.

2. Mix in vanilla yogurt, honey, and vanilla extract.

3. Combine until thoroughly combined.

4. Before serving, let the food cool for half an hour in the fridge.

Guidelines:

Bananas are mild on the digestive system and contain potassium, while yogurt contains probiotics that promote intestinal health.

2. APPLESAUCE CAKE

INGREDIENTS:

• One cup of unsweetened applesauce

• One cup of sugar

• 1/2 cup of vegetable oil

• Two eggs

• Two cups of flour

• One teaspoon of baking soda

• One teaspoon of cinnamon

STEPS:

1. Set the oven's temperature to 175°C/350°F.

2. Combine oil, sugar, and applesauce in a sizable basin.

3. Incorporate the eggs.

4. Gradually incorporate cinnamon, baking soda, and flour, ensuring that they are thoroughly combined.

5. Pour the batter into a baking tin that has been greased.

6. 30 to 35 minutes or until a probe is removed spotless.

7. Let cool completely before serving.

Guidelines:

Applesauce is an excellent low-fiber fruit substitute that contributes moisture to the cake and facilitates digestion.

3. RICE PUDDING

INGREDIENTS:

• One cup of white rice

• Two glasses of milk

- One-half cup of sugar

- One teaspoon of vanilla extract

- 1/4 teaspoon of dried cinnamon

STEPS:

1. Prepare rice by the manufacturer's instructions.

2. Combine cooked rice, milk, sugar, and vanilla extract in a saucepan.

3. Stir the mixture frequently over medium heat until it becomes viscous and creamy.

4. Before serving, sprinkle with powdered cinnamon.

Guidelines:

White rice is an appropriate choice for an ileostomy diet due to its minimal fiber content and gentle digestion.

INGREDIENTS:

• One package of lemon-flavored gelatin

• One cup of simmering water

• One cup of lukewarm water

STEPS:

1. Boiling water is used to dissolve gelatin.

2. Incorporate frigid water and agitate thoroughly.

3. Pour the mixture into molds and refrigerate until it has solidified.

Guidelines:

Gelatin desserts are ideal for individuals with sensitive digestive systems, as they are both light and simple to ingest.

5. CUSTARD THAT HAS BEEN BAKED

INGREDIENTS:

• Two glasses of milk

• Three eggs

• One-half cup of sugar

• One teaspoon of vanilla extract

• A small amount of nutmeg

STEPS:

1. Set oven temperature to 325°F, or 160°C.

2. Heat the milk until it is tepid, but not scalding.

3. Whisk together sugar, vanilla extract, and eggs in a basin.

4. Stir continuously, and gradually incorporate heated milk into the egg mixture.

5. Transfer the mixture to ramekins.

6. Place the ramekins in a baking dish and pour hot water into the dish until it reaches midway up the sides of the ramekins.

7. Until the custard is completely set, bake for 40-45 minutes.

8. Before serving, sprinkle with nutmeg.

Guidelines:

Baked custard is a nutritious source of calcium and protein that is not too taxing on the digestive system.

6. SMOOTHIE POPSICLES

INGREDIENTS:

• One cup of strawberry yogurt

• One-half cup of milk

• One banana

• One tablespoon of honey

STEPS:

1. All ingredients should be blended until they are homogeneous.

2. Pour the mixture into popsicle molds.

3. Freeze until it becomes solid, which should take approximately 4-6 hours.

Guidelines:

These popsicles are both invigorating and easily digestible, as they combine the advantages of bananas and yogurt.

7. VANILLA RICE PUDDING

INGREDIENTS:

• Arborio rice, 1/2 cup

• Four glasses of milk

• 1/4 cup of sugar

• One teaspoon of vanilla extract

• 1/4 teaspoon of dried cinnamon

STEPS:

1. Rice and milk should be combined in a saucepan.

2. Bring the mixture to a boil, then reduces the heat and allows it to simmer, stirring occasionally, until the rice is tender and the pudding is dense.

3. Stir in vanilla extract and sugar.

4. Before serving, sprinkle with powdered cinnamon.

Guidelines:

Arborio rice is a soothing dessert option for ileostomy patients, as it is creamy and simpler to ingest.

General Recommendations For An Ileostomy Diet:

1. Low Fiber: Emphasize low-fiber foods to prevent blockages. It is recommended that fruits and vegetables be peeled and cooked to reduce their fiber content.

2. Hydration is crucial, as fluid loss may be exacerbated by an ileostomy.

3. Thoroughly chew: To facilitate digestion, ensure that you consume the food thoroughly.

4. Refrain from Consuming High-Fat Foods: Consuming high-fat foods can result in digestive issues and discomfort.

5. Introduce New Foods Gradually: To assess tolerance, incorporate new foods into your diet one at a time.

6. Small, Frequent Meals: Consume smaller, more frequent meals to facilitate digestion.

7. Continue to engage in gentle physical activity, as it can enhance digestion and overall health.

These delicacies and guidelines offer a balanced approach to consuming treats while adhering to a diet that is appropriate for an ileostomy. Take care of your digestive health while indulging in these delectable delights!

CHAPTER FOURTEEN

Seven Smoothies For An Ileostomy Diet: Recipes And Recommendations

It can be somewhat more difficult for individuals who are living with an ileostomy to maintain a balanced diet. Smoothies are an exceptional choice due to their versatility, ease of digestion, and potential for nutrient denseness. Below are seven smoothie recipes that are specifically designed for an ileostomy diet, with an emphasis on ingredients that are readily digestible and minimal in residue.

Smoothies in an ileostomy diet should adhere to the following guidelines:

1. Low-Fiber Ingredients: Select fruits and vegetables that are low in fiber to prevent blockages. Steer clear of seeds, shells, and fibers.

2. Hydration: To guarantee sufficient hydration, consume liquids such as coconut water, water, or lactose-free milk.

3. Nutrient Balance: To preserve nutritional equilibrium, incorporate protein sources such as protein powder or yogurt.

4. Avoid Gassy Ingredients: Avoid cruciferous vegetables (e.g., broccoli, cabbage) and other ingredients that may induce flatulence.

5. fluid Texture: Guarantee that all ingredients are thoroughly incorporated to a fluid consistency to facilitate digestion.

6. Sugar Moderation: To prevent excessive sugar consumption, employ natural sweeteners such as honey or dates sparingly.

1. SMOOTHIE WITH BLUEBERRIES AND BANANAS

INGREDIENTS:

• One mature banana

• 1/2 cup of blueberries, either fresh or frozen

• One cup of almond milk or lactose-free milk

• One-half cup of Greek yogurt

• One tablespoon of honey

DIRECTIONS:

1. Slice the banana after it has been peeled.

2. In a blender, combine the banana, blueberries, milk, Greek yogurt, and honey.

3. Blend until the mixture is uniform.

4. Serve immediately.

INGREDIENTS:

• One cup of pineapple chunks (drained, whether fresh or canned)

• 1/2 cup of mango chunks (fresh or frozen)

• One cup of coconut water

• One-half cup of plain yogurt

• One tablespoon of maple syrup

DIRECTIONS:

1. In a blender, combine the yogurt, maple syrup, pineapple, mango, and coconut water.

2. Blend until the mixture is entirely smooth.

3. Pour the beverage into a glass and savor it.

3. SMOOTHIE WITH PEACHES AND KEFIR

INGREDIENTS:

• One cup of cut peaches (fresh or tinned, drained)

• 1/2 cup of kefir (lactose-free if necessary)

• One-half cup of citrus juice

• 1 tablespoon of chia seeds (optional; marinate for 10 minutes)

• One teaspoon of vanilla extract

DIRECTIONS:

1. To a blender, combine the soaked chia seeds, orange juice, kefir, and vanilla extract. Add the peaches.

2. Blend until the mixture is velvety and smooth.

3. Chill before serving.

INGREDIENTS:

• 1 cup of cubed honeydew melon

• One cup of cubed melons

• 1/2 cup of almond milk or lactose-free milk

• 1/2 cup of ice crystals

• 5 fresh mint fronds

• One teaspoon of honey (optional)

DIRECTIONS:

1. Melon cubes, milk, ice cubes, mint sprigs, and honey should be combined in a blender.

2. Blend until the mixture is frothy and smooth.

3. Pour the mixture into a glass and serve.

INGREDIENTS:

• One mature avocado, skinned and pitted

• One mature banana

• One cup of almond milk or lactose-free milk

• One-half cup of vanilla yogurt

• One tablespoon of honey

DIRECTIONS:

1. Combine banana, avocado, yogurt, milk, and honey in a Vitamix.

2. Blend until the mixture is smooth and velvety.

3. For optimal flavor, serve immediately.

6. SMOOTHIE WITH STRAWBERRIES AND BANANAS

INGREDIENTS:

• One cup of hulled strawberries, either fresh or preserved

• One mature banana

• One cup of almond milk or lactose-free milk

• One-half cup of Greek yogurt

• One tablespoon of agave syrup

DIRECTIONS:

1. Combine strawberries, bananas, milk, Greek yogurt, and agave nectar in a Vitamix.

2. Blend until the mixture is uniform.

3. Pour the beverage into a glass and savor it.

INGREDIENTS:

• One cup of unsweetened applesauce

• 1/2 cup of almond milk or lactose-free milk

• One-half cup of vanilla yogurt

• 1/2 teaspoon granulated cinnamon

• One tablespoon of maple syrup

DIRECTIONS:

1. Place applesauce, milk, yogurt, cinnamon, and maple syrup in a Vitamix.

2. Blend until well combined and smooth.

3. Serve refrigerated or at room temperature.

General Tips:

• Experiment with Flavors: Feel free to mix and match the ingredients to suit your flavor while maintaining within the dietary guidelines.

• Storage: Smoothies are best ingested fresh, but they can be stored in the refrigerator for up to 24 hours. Stir well before consuming.

• Hydration Boost: Adding a few ice crystals can make the smoothies more refreshing, particularly in warmer weather.

These beverages are designed to be simple on the digestive system while providing essential nutrients and hydration. They are ideal for anyone seeking to maintain a balanced diet after ileostomy surgery. Enjoy the variety and health benefits these beverages offer!

CHAPTER FIFTEEN

Dining Out And Social Situations

Eating out can be daunting for individuals with an ileostomy, but with some savvy tactics, it can be enjoyable and stress-free. Ensure that you review the menu online in advance to identify secure choices, such as grilled chicken or seafood, steamed vegetables, and rice. Do not hesitate to inform the server of your dietary restrictions when placing an order.

For instance, to regulate one's consumption, it is advisable to request condiments and dressings on the side and steer clear of dishes that are excessively oily or spicy, as They could cause upset stomachs. If the primary dishes appear to be excessively large, consider ordering lesser portions or appetizers.

In the event of an emergency, it is advisable to discreetly transport a small supply of ostomy supplies in your purse. Do not allow your ileostomy to restrict your social life; rather, employ these strategies to confidently navigate dining out.

It is essential to be prepared with portable meals and refreshment options to manage appetite and maintain energy levels throughout the day. For on-the-go snacks, bring foods that are easily digestible, such as bananas, yogurt, rice cakes, and nut butter sachets.

For meals, contemplate constructing sandwiches with soft, readily digestible fillings, such as scrambled eggs or tuna salad. Pre-cut fruits and vegetables, such as carrots, pears, and cucumber segments, are both nutritious and convenient. Invest in a quality insulated picnic bag to keep perishable items fresh, and always carry extra ostomy supplies just in case.

These portable alternatives enable you to sustain a nutritious diet and remain content regardless of your daily activities.

Tips For Eating Out Safely

It is essential to prioritize food safety when dining out to prevent potential complications with your ileostomy. Select establishments that are known for their clean facilities and their commitment to the proper management of food. When placing an order, prioritize dishes that are readily digestible and well-cooked, such as grilled or baked proteins, steamed vegetables, and simple rice or pasta.

It is advisable to steer clear of raw or undercooked foods, as they may be more difficult to digest and may increase the likelihood of bacterial contamination. Please notify your server of your dietary restrictions and inquire about the ingredients or preparation methods if you are uncertain. You can dine out safely and worry-free by being proactive and selective in your choices.

A strategic approach is necessary to ensure optimal digestion and minimal distress when navigating restaurant menus with an ileostomy. Making smart menu choices are essential. Select menu items that are low in fiber and cholesterol, as these can be more difficult to digest and may result in digestive issues.

Select lean protein sources, such as chicken, fish, or tofu, and combine them with basic carbohydrates, such as rice or potatoes, and well-cooked vegetables.

Dishes that contain hefty sauces, spicy seasonings, or excessive quantities of dairy should be avoided, as they may exacerbate digestive symptoms.

Alternatively, select seared or steamed dishes and request that they be adjusted to accommodate your dietary requirements. You can savor delectable meals without sacrificing your digestive health by making informed menu selections.

It is imperative to effectively communicate your dietary requirements to restaurant personnel, friends, and family to guarantee a comfortable dining experience with an ileostomy. Be forthright and forthright regarding your dietary restrictions, providing a rationale for your decisions if required.

It is crucial to provide loved ones with explicit instructions when they are preparing meals, emphasizing the significance of avoiding trigger foods or ingredients. Do not hesitate to inquire about the menu options or request modifications to suit your requirements when dining out. A dietary card or note that outlines your restrictions should be carried with you to present to stewards or chefs if necessary. You can confidently navigate social situations and appreciate meals without concern by communicating assertively and advocating for yourself.

Conclusion

Individuals with an ileostomy need to adhere to an ileostomy diet to maintain optimal health and prevent complications. The primary goal of this regimen is to prevent blockages, minimize discomfort, and manage and control the outflow of the stoma.

Initially, patients are advised to adhere to a low-fiber diet to mitigate the risk of intestinal obstructions and facilitate the digestive system's adaptation.

Individuals can progressively reintroduce higher-fiber foods as their bodies acclimate over time.

The ileostomy can increase fluid loss, so it is important to stay hydrated. Additionally, consuming smaller, more frequent meals can help facilitate digestion. Nuts, seeds, and raw vegetables are foods that are known to cause blockages, and it is crucial to chew them thoroughly and avoid them.

Foods that may induce excessive flatulence or odor, such as legumes, cruciferous vegetables, and carbonated beverages, should be consumed in moderation or avoided altogether.

It is crucial to monitor the impact of various substances on the stoma output and overall comfort of each individual, as their tolerance varies.

The diet can be customized to meet the specific requirements of the individual, thereby enhancing the quality of life and assuring balanced nutrition, by collaborating closely with a healthcare provider or dietitian.

Individuals with an ileostomy can effectively manage their condition and maintain a healthy lifestyle by adhering to these dietary guidelines.

THE END

www.ingramcontent.com/pod-product-compliance
Lightning Source LLC
Chambersburg PA
CBHW052318220526
45472CB00001B/173